Vegetarian Cookbook

The Best Recipes to Eat Vegetarian At Every Meal

By
Linda Parker

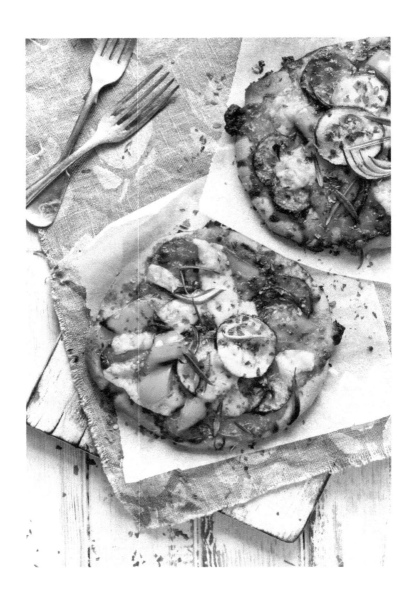

that may befall them after undertaking information
described herein.

Additionally, the information in the following pages is
intended only for informational purposes and should thus
be thought of as universal. As befitting its nature, it is
presented without assurance regarding its prolonged
validity or interim quality. Trademarks that are mentioned
are done without written consent and can in no way be
considered an endorsement from the trademark holder.

Table of Contents

Introduction

Vegetarianism refers to a lifestyle that excludes the consumption of all forms of meat including pork, chicken, beef, lamb, venison, fish, and shells. Depending on a person's belief and lifestyle, vegetarianism has different spectrums. There are vegetarians, who like to consume products that come from animals such as milk, eggs, cream and cheese. On the other end of that spectrum are the vegans. Vegans never consume meat or any product that comes from animals.

Benefits of Vegetarianism

According to research, living a vegetarian lifestyle lowers your risk of getting some of the major chronic diseases such as heart disease, cancer and type 2 diabetes. Vegetarians are 19 to 25% less likely to die of any kind of heart disease. The high consumption of fiber from grains also prevents the blood sugar spikes that lead to heart attacks and diabetes. The consumption of nuts, which are high in fiber, antioxidants and omega 3 fatty acids also helps lower the vegetarian's risk of getting heart attacks.

Due to the avoidance of red meat, you'll also eliminate a great deal of risk in getting certain types of cancer such as colon cancer. The high level of antioxidants from green leafy vegetables and fruits also helps in this area.

What About These Missing Nutrients?

Some people may be concerned with the lack of the following nutrients in a vegetarian diet however you'll find that there are certain types of vegetables and fruits that can supply these nutrients to give you a perfectly balanced diet. Some of the nutrients of concern are protein, iron, calcium and vitamin b12.

Protein can easily be found in beans and products made from beans such as tofu. Nuts and peas are also good sources of protein. Iron can also be found in tofu, beans, spinach, chard and cashews. Calcium can easily be found in soy milk, broccoli, collard greens, mustard greens and kale.

How to Make The Change

When you're starting out with this lifestyle, you might want to take baby steps. Start with 1 vegetarian meal per day. This allows you to adapt gradually to the different taste and flavors of a vegetarian diet. Once you're used to having a vegetarian meal every day, you can slowly add one more vegetarian meal until you've completely changed your lifestyle. Research has found that making small changes is more sustainable in the end. It's not a contest. Take your time and enjoy the different types of vegetarian meals. How To Use This Book As you browse through the pages, figure out which recipes you like and make them a part of your daily life. This book is filled with different types of vegan dishes and some of them include classic dishes that have been adapted to suit the vegan diet.

BREAKFAST

Ultimate Breakfast Sandwich

Preparation time: 40 minutes
Cooking time: 10 minutes
Servings: 4

Ingredients:

For the Tofu:

- 12 ounces tofu, extra-firm, pressed, drain
- 1/2 teaspoon garlic powder
- 1 teaspoon liquid smoke
- 2 tablespoons nutritional yeast
- 1 teaspoon Sriracha sauce
- 2 tablespoons soy sauce
- 2 tablespoons olive oil
- 2 tablespoons water

For the Vegan Breakfast Sandwich:

- 1 large tomato, sliced
- 4 English muffins, halved, toasted
- 1 avocado, mashed

Directions:

1. Prepare tofu, and for this, cut tofu into four slices and set aside.

2. Stir together remaining ingredients of tofu, pour the mixture into a bag, then add tofu pieces, toss until coated and marinate for 30 minutes.
3. Take a skillet pan, place it over medium-high heat, add tofu slices along with the marinade and cook for 5 minutes per side.
4. Prepare the sandwich and for this, spread mashed avocado on the inner of the muffin, top with a slice of tofu, layer with a tomato slice and then serve.

Pancake

Preparation time: 10 minutes
Cooking time: 18 minutes
Servings: 4

Ingredients:
Dry Ingredients:
- 1 cup buckwheat flour
- 1/8 teaspoon salt
- ½ teaspoon gluten-free baking powder
- ½ teaspoon baking soda

Wet Ingredients:
- 1 tablespoon almond butter
- 2 tablespoon maple syrup
- 1 tablespoon lime juice
- 1 cup coconut milk, unsweetened

Directions:
1. Take a medium bowl, add all the dry ingredients and stir until mixed.
2. Take another bowl, place all the wet ingredients, whisk until combined, and then gradually whisk in dry ingredients mixture until smooth and incorporated.
3. Take a frying pan, place it over medium heat, add 2 teaspoons oil and when hot, drop in batter and cook

for 3 minutes per side until cooked and lightly browned.
4. Serve pancakes and fruits and maple syrup.

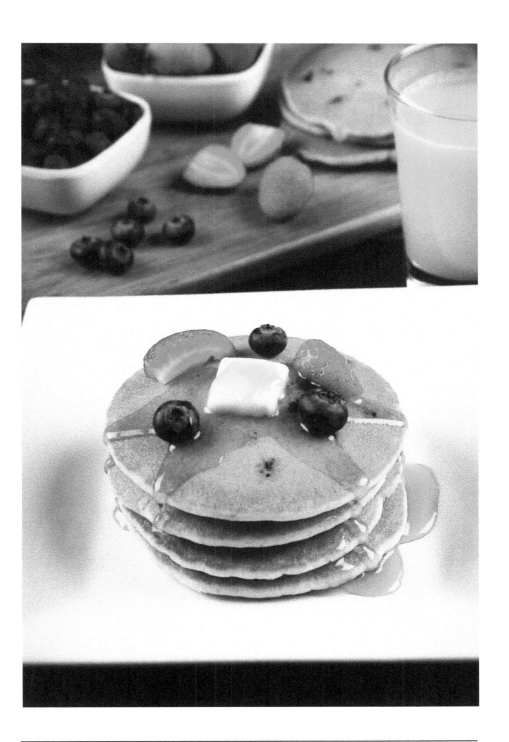

Herb & Cheese Omelet

Preparation Time: 5 minutes
Cooking Time: 5 minutes
Servings: 2

Ingredients:
- 4 eggs Salt and pepper to taste
- 2 tbsp. low-fat milk
- 1 tsp. chives, chopped 1 tbsp. parsley, chopped
- ½ cup goat cheese, crumbled
- 1 tsp. olive oil

Directions:
1. Beat the eggs in a bowl.
2. Stir in the salt, pepper and milk.
3. In a bowl, combine the chives, parsley and goat cheese.
4. Pour the oil into a pan over medium heat.
5. Cook the eggs for 3 minutes.
6. Add the cheese mixture on top.
7. Fold and serve.

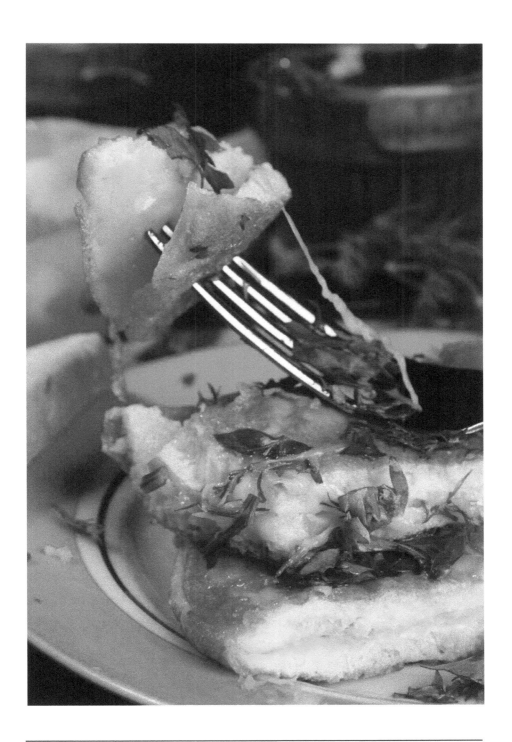

Green Breakfast Salad

Preparation Time: 10 minutes
Cooking time: 10 minutes
Servings: 4

Ingredients:
- 1 tablespoon lemon juice
- 4 red bell peppers
- 1 lettuce head, cut into strips
- Salt and black pepper to the taste
- 3 tablespoons coconut cream
- 2 tablespoons olive oil
- 1 ounces rocket leaves

Directions:
1. Place bell pepper in your air fryer's basket, cook at 400 degrees F for 10 minutes, transfer to a bowl, leave them aside to cool down, peel, cut them in strips and put them in a bowl.
2. Add rocket leaves and lettuce strips and toss.
3. In a bowl, mix oil with lemon juice, coconut cream, salt and pepper, whisk well, add over the salad, toss to coat, divide between plates and serve for breakfast.
4. Enjoy!

Wheat Quick Bread

Servings: 1 loaf
Preparation Time: 10 mins
Cooking Time: 20 mins

Ingredients:

- 1 cup rolled oats
- 1 cup whole wheat flour
- 1 cup soy milk
- 2 tsp. baking powder
- 1½ tbsp. agave syrup
- 1 tbsp. vegetable oil
- 1 tsp. salt

Directions:

1. Preheat the oven to 450 degrees Fahrenheit.
2. In a food processor or blender, grind the oatmeal to make oatmeal flour.
3. Combine oatmeal flour, whole wheat flour, baking powder and salt.
4. In a separate bowl, dissolve the agave syrup in vegetable oil, and then stir in the soy milk.
5. Combine both the dry and wet mixtures and stir until they form a soft dough.
6. Form the dough into a smooth round ball and place on a lightly oiled baking sheet.

7. Bake it for 20 minutes, or until the bottom crust of loaf sounds hollow when tapped.

Sweet Pomegranate Porridge

Preparation time: 5 minutes
Cooking time: 30 minutes
Servings: 4

Ingredients:
- 2 Cups Oats
- 1 ½ Cups Water
- 1 ½ Cups Pomegranate Juice
- 2 Tablespoons Pomegranate Molasses

Directions:
1. Pour all ingredients into the instant pot and mix well.
2. Seal the lid, and cook on high pressure for four minutes.
3. Use a quick release, and serve warm.

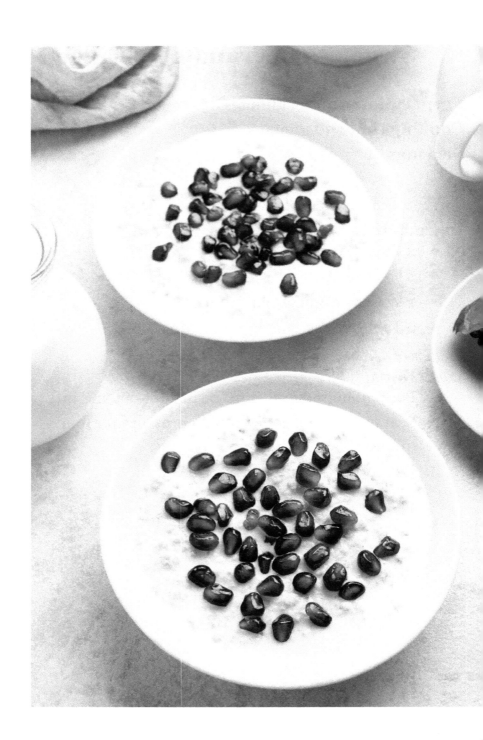

Potato and Zucchini Omelet

Preparation time: 5 minutes
Cooking time: 20 minutes

Ingredients:
- ½ lb. potato (about 1¼ cups diced)
- ½ lb. zucchini (about 1½ cups diced)
- ⅔ cup chopped onion (1 small)
- 1 Tbs. butter
- 2 Tbsp. olive oil
- ¼ tsp. dried dill weed
- ¼ tsp. dried basil, crushed
- ½ tsp. crushed dried red pepper
- salt to taste
- fresh-ground black pepper to taste
- 5 to 6 eggs
- butter for frying
- garnish sour cream

Directions:
1. Peel or scrub the potato and cut it in ½-inch dice.
2. Wash, trim, and finely dice the zucchini.
3. Drop the diced potato into boiling salted water and cook for 5 minutes, then drain it and set it aside.
4. Cook the diced zucchini in boiling water for 3 to 4 minutes, drain, and set aside.

5. Heat the butter and the olive oil in a medium-sized skillet and sauté the onions in it until they start to color.
6. Add the partially cooked potato and zucchini, the dill weed, basil, crushed red pepper, and salt.
7. Cook this mixture over medium heat, stirring often, until the potatoes are just tender.
8. Grind in some black pepper and add more salt if needed.
9. Make either 2 medium-sized or 3 small omelets according to the directions.
10. When the eggs are almost set, spoon some of the hot vegetables onto one side and fold the other side of the omelet over the filling.
11. Slide the omelets out onto warm plates and serve immediately with sour cream.

Tomato Omelet

Preparation time: 5 minutes
Cooking time: 40 minutes
Servings: 3

Ingredients:

- 8 medium sized tomatoes
- 2 cloves garlic
- 2 bay leaves
- ½ tsp. dried tarragon, crushed
- 1 tsp. salt, and more to taste
- 2 Tbsp. chopped fresh parsley
- 1 medium sized yellow onion
- 3 Tbs. olive oil
- ½ tsp. dried basil, crushed
- 5 cured black olives, pitted and sliced coarse
- ground black pepper to taste
- 8 to 10 eggs
- milk

Directions:
1. Blanch the tomatoes in boiling water for about 2 minutes and then peel them.
2. Chop the tomatoes very coarsely and put them aside in a bowl with the salt.

3. Chop the onion, mince the garlic, and sauté them in the olive oil in a large skillet until they begin to show color.
4. Add the bay leaves and sauté a few minutes more.
5. Add the tomatoes, the basil, tarragon, parsley, and sliced olives, and cook over medium heat, stirring occasionally, until the sauce is thick.
6. It should take about 40 to 45 minutes.
7. Make individual omelets according to the directions.
8. Spoon on some of the hot Provençale sauce just when the eggs are nearly set.
9. Serve.

Vegan Tropical Pina Colada Smoothie

Preparation time: 5 minutes
Cooking time: 0 minutes
Servings: 1 smoothie

Ingredients:

- ¾ cup soymilk
- ½ cup coconut milk
- 1 banana
- 1 ½ tbsp. ground flaxseed
- 1 tsp. vanilla
- 1 cup pineapple
- 1 tbsp. agave nectar
- 3 ice cubes

Directions:

1. Bring all the above ingredients together in a blender, and blend the ingredients to achieve your desired smoothie consistency.
2. Enjoy!

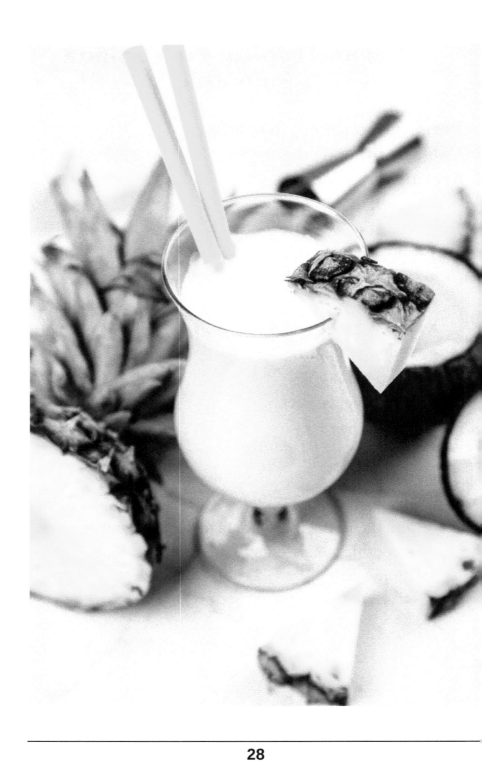

Peach Protein Bars

Servings: 6
Preparation Time: 60 min

Ingredients:
- 1 cup flax seeds
- ½ cup peanuts
- ¼ cup hemp seeds
- 15g dehydrated peaches
- 2 tbsp. psyllium husk
- ¼ tsp. stevia
- ½ tsp. salt
- 1¼ cup water

Total number of Ingredients: 8

Directions:
1. Preheat the oven at 350°F.
2. Grind up nuts and seeds with ½ cup water in a blender, but make sure the mixture is not finely ground.
3. Transfer and combine mixture with psyllium husk and cinnamon in a mixing bowl.
4. Crush the dehydrated peaches into small bits and add to the mixing bowl.

5. Stir in the remaining water and salt until all Ingredients are combined.
6. Let the mixture sit for a few minutes.
7. Spread the mixture out on a baking sheet lined with parchment paper, and make sure the dough is about ¼ inch thick.
8. Bake for 45 minutes, remove around 30 minutes to cut the dough carefully in six pieces, and bake for another 15 minutes.
9. Remove from the oven and cool for 30 minutes.
10. Can be stored for a week or frozen up to two months.

Breakfast Tacos

Preparation Time: 10 minutes
Cooking time: 6 minutes
Servings: 4

Ingredients:
- ½ cup grape tomatoes, quartered
- 1 avocado, sliced
- 8 corn tortillas
- Freshly ground black pepper
- ¼ teaspoon salt
- ¼ teaspoon cumin
- ¼ teaspoon ground turmeric
- 1 package firm tofu
- 1 garlic clove, minced
- 1 red pepper, diced
- 1 teaspoon olive oil

Directions:
1. Heat oil in a skillet over medium heat.
2. Add in garlic and red pepper and sauté for around 2 minutes.
3. Using your hands, crumble the tofu and add into the pan; and then add the seasonings.
4. Cook for around 5 minutes making sure that you stir frequently.

5. Taste and adjust the seasonings then apportion it and store in containers for the week.
6. When you want to serve, simply put the scramble on tortillas, add any other toppings and enjoy.

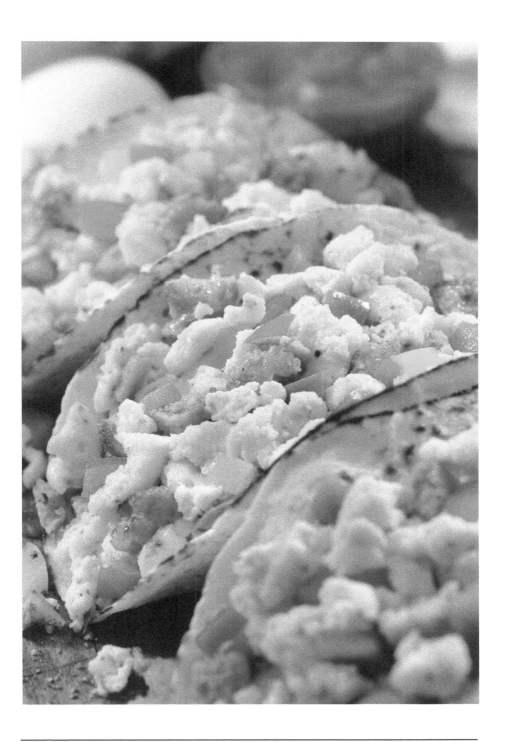

Breakfast Cookies

Preparation Time: 10 minutes
Cooking time: 6 minutes
Servings: Makes 24-32

Ingredients:
Dry Ingredients

- ½ teaspoon baking powder
- 2 cups rolled oats
- ½ teaspoon baking soda

Wet Ingredients

- 1 teaspoon pure vanilla extract
- 2 flax eggs
- 2 tablespoons ground flaxseed and around
- 6 tablespoons of water, mix and put aside for 15 minutes
- 2 tablespoons melted coconut oil
- 2 tablespoons pure maple syrup
- ½ cup natural creamy peanut butter
- 2 ripe bananas

Add-in Ingredients

- ½ cup finely chopped walnuts
- ½ cup raisins

Optional Topping

- 2 tablespoons chopped walnuts

- 2 tablespoons raisins

Directions:
1. Preheat the oven to 325 degrees F, and then use parchment paper to line a baking sheet and put aside.
2. Add the bananas in a large bowl, and then use a fork to mash them until smooth.
3. Add in the other wet Ingredients and mix until well incorporated.
4. Add the dry Ingredients and then use a rubber spatula to stir and fold them into the dry Ingredients until well mixed.
5. Stir in the walnuts and raisins.
6. Scoop the cookie dough onto the prepared baking sheet making sure that you leave adequate space between the cookies.
7. Bake in the preheated oven for around 12 minutes.
8. Once ready, let the cookies cool on the baking sheet for around 10 minutes.
9. Lift the cookies carefully from the baking sheet onto a cooling rack to further cool.
10. Store the cookies in an airtight container in the fridge or at room temperature for up to one week.

SOUPS

Watercress and Carrot Soup

Ingredients:
- 1 tablespoon sesame oil
- 3 teaspoons crushed garlic
- 1 tablespoon chopped fresh cilantro
- 2 teaspoons chili garlic sauce
- 1 red onion, chopped
- 3 large carrots, peeled and sliced
- 1 bunch watercress, coarsely chopped
- 5 cups vegetable stock

Directions:
1. Heat oil in a pot over medium heat.
2. Cook garlic, cilantro and chili garlic sauce.
3. Cook onions until tender.
4. Add the carrots and watercress.
5. Cook for 5 minutes and pour in vegetable stock.
6. Simmer for 40 minutes, or until spinach and carrots become soft.
7. Blend until smooth.

Thai Turnip and Sweet Potato Soup

Ingredients:
- 1 tablespoon sesame seed oil
- 3 teaspoons crushed garlic
- 1 tablespoon chopped fresh cilantro
- 1 teaspoon Thai bird chilies, minced
- 2 tbsp. tamarind paste
- 1 tsp. Thai chili paste
- 1 red onion, chopped
- 3 large turnips, peeled and sliced
- 1 large sweet potato, peeled and chopped
- 5 cups vegetable broth

Directions:
1. Heat oil in a pot over medium heat.
2. Cook garlic, cilantro, Thai chilies, tamarind paste, and Thai chili paste.
3. Cook onions until tender.
4. Add the turnips and potato.
5. Cook for 5 minutes and pour in vegetable stock.
6. Simmer for 40 minutes, or until potatoes and turnips become soft.
7. Blend until smooth.

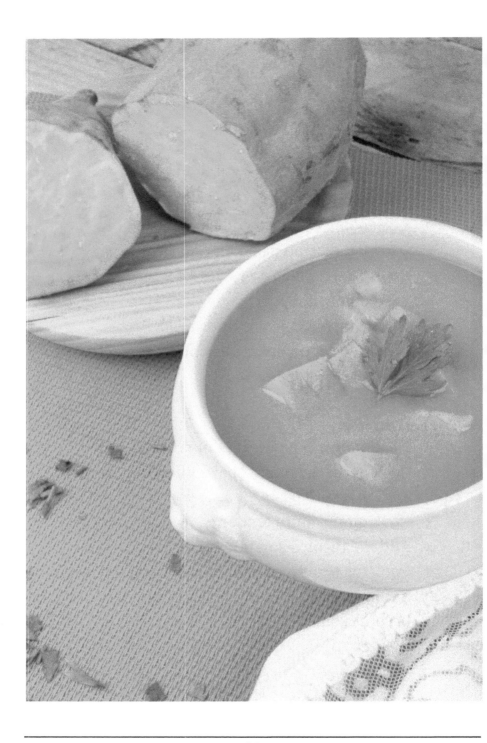

Summer Squash and Lemon Grass Soup

Ingredients:
- 1 tablespoon extra-virgin olive oil
- 3 teaspoons crushed garlic
- 1 tablespoon chopped fresh cilantro
- 2 to 3 stalks lemongrass
- 1 tsp. ginger, finely minced
- 1 red onion, chopped
- 3 large summer squash, peeled and sliced
- 1 large potato, peeled and chopped
- 5 cups vegetable stock

Directions:
1. Heat oil in a pot over medium heat.
2. Cook garlic, cilantro, lemon grass,& ginger.
3. Cook onions until tender.
4. Add the squash and potato.
5. Cook for 5 minutes and pour in vegetable stock.
6. Simmer for 40 minutes, or until potatoes and squash become soft.
7. Blend until smooth.

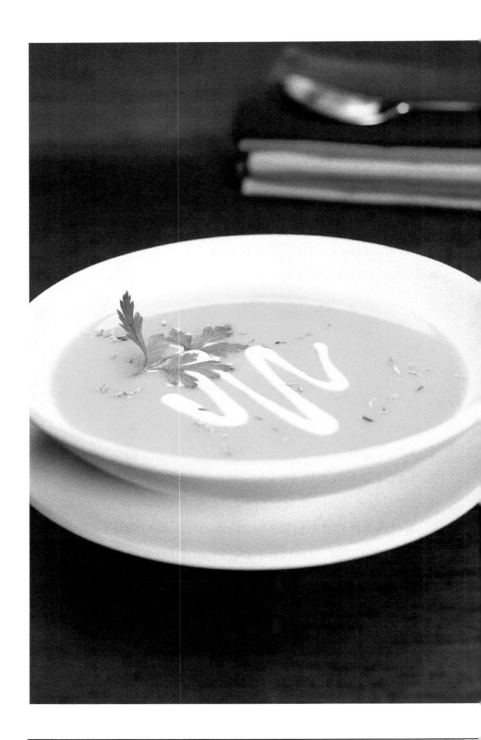

Summer Squash and Winter Soup

Ingredients:
- 1 tablespoon sesame seed oil
- 7 teaspoons crushed garlic
- 1 tablespoon chopped fresh cilantro
- 1 teaspoon Chinese five spice powder
- 1 teaspoon chili garlic paste
- 1 red onion, chopped
- 3 large pcs. of summer squash, peeled and sliced
- 1 large winter squash, peeled and chopped
- 5 cups vegetable broth

Directions:
1. Heat oil in a pot over medium heat.
2. Cook garlic, cilantro and chili paste.
3. Cook onions until tender.
4. Add the squash.
5. Cook for 5 minutes and pour in vegetable stock.
6. Simmer for 40 minutes, or until squash becomes soft.
7. Blend until smooth.

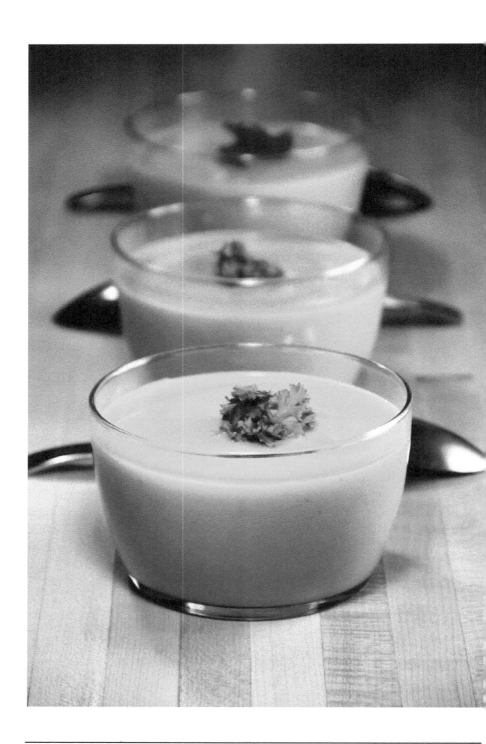

Creamy Parsnip and Peanut Soup

Poblano Soup

Ingredients:
- 4 tablespoons salted butter
- 1 small red onion, coarsely chopped
- 1 large leek, white part only, sliced
- 1 green bell pepper, coarsely chopped
- 5 pcs. Thai chilies, sliced
- 5 Thai basil leaves
- 2 tbsp. tamarind paste
- 8 cloves garlic, diced
- 1 large parsnip, cubed (you can use two if you like your soup thick)
- 4 cups vegetable broth
- 1 cup peanuts
- 1-1/4 coconut milk
- Sea salt
- Black pepper

Directions:
Optional garnish:
1. Sliced jalapeno pepper.
2. Soak peanuts in almond milk for an hour.
3. Melt non-dairy butter in a pan.

4. Add the red onion, leek, chilies, Thai basil, tamarind paste, bell pepper, garlic, and potato.
5. Cook on low heat and stir until the onion is translucent, 6 1/2 minutes.
6. Add the broth into the pan.
7. Simmer until the parsnips are fork tender for about 25 minutes.
8. Take it off the heat.
9. Process the mixture in a blender until smooth.
10. Return the soup to the pan. In the blender, blend peanuts with coconut milk until smooth.
11. Add to the soup mixture.
12. Heat the soup on medium heat for a few more minutes.
13. Garnish with slices of jalapeno.

Lentil and Butternut Squash Curry Soup

Ingredients:
- 1 tablespoon sesame seed oil
- 1 small red onion, chopped
- 1 tablespoon minced fresh ginger root
- 3 cloves garlic, chopped
- 1 pinch fenugreek seeds
- 1 cup dry red lentils
- 1 cup butternut squash - peeled, seeded, and cubed
- 1/3 cup finely chopped fresh cilantro
- 2 cups water
- 1/2 (14 ounce) can almond milk
- 2 tablespoons tomato paste
- 1 teaspoon red curry powder
- 1/4 cayenne pepper
- 1 pinch ground nutmeg
- salt and pepper to taste

Directions:
1. Heat the oil in a pot over medium heat.
2. Sauté the onion, garlic, and fenugreek until the onion becomes tender.
3. Add the lentils, squash, and cilantro into the pot.
4. Add the water, almond milk, and tomato paste.
5. Season with curry powder, cayenne pepper, nutmeg, salt, and pepper.

6. Boil and reduce heat to low Simmer until lentils and squash are tender for about 30 min.

Thai Curried Butternut Squash Soup

Ingredients:
- 1 tablespoon sesame seed oil
- 1 small red onion, chopped
- 1 tablespoon minced fresh ginger root
- 3 cloves garlic, chopped
- 1 cup peanuts
- 1 cup butternut squash - peeled, seeded, and cubed
- 1/3 cup finely chopped fresh cilantro
- 2 cups water
- 1/2 (14 ounce) can coconut milk
- 1 teaspoon red curry powder
- 1tsp. Thai bird chilies
- 1 pinch ground nutmeg
- salt and pepper to taste

Directions:
1. Heat the oil in a pot over medium heat.
2. Sauté the onion, ginger, and garlic until the onion becomes tender.
3. Add the peanuts, squash, and cilantro into the pot.
4. Add the water & coconut milk.
5. Season with curry powder, Thai bird chilies, nutmeg, salt, and pepper.
6. Boil and reduce heat to low.
7. Simmer until peanuts and squash are tender for about 30 min.

Simple Carrot and Tarragon Soup

Ingredients:
- 2 tablespoons extra virgin olive oil
- 1 small red onion, minced
- 1 medium carrot, peeled and thinly sliced
- 1 celery rib, thinly sliced
- 1/2 teaspoon dried tarragon
- 2 cups vegetable stock
- 1/4 cup wine vinegar

Directions:
1. Heat the oil over medium-high heat.
2. Sauté red onions until tender for about 5 minutes.
3. Slowly add carrots, celery, and tarragon.
4. Cook for another 5 minutes, or until carrots become tender.
5. Add vegetable broth and vinegar Boil and simmer.
6. Cook for 15 minutes longer.

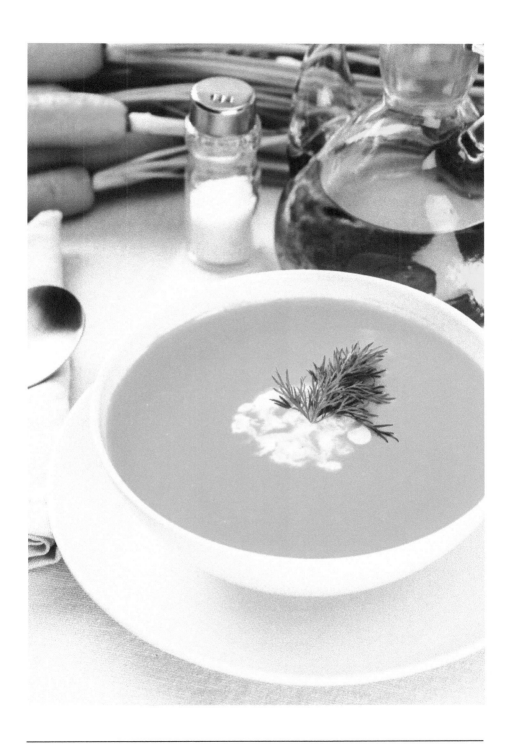

Thai Carrot Soup

Ingredients:
- 2 tablespoons sesame seed oil
- 1 small red onion, minced
- 1 small carrot, peeled and thinly sliced
- 1/2 teaspoon Thai chili paste
- 2 cups vegetable broth
- 1/4 cup coconut or white vinegar
- 1 sprig cilantro

Directions:
1. Heat the oil over medium-high heat.
2. Sauté red onions until tender for about 5 minutes.
3. Slowly add carrots and chili paste.
4. Cook for another 5 minutes, or until carrots become tender.
5. Add vegetable stock and vinegar.
6. Boil and simmer.
7. Cook for 15 minutes longer.

Hungarian Carrot Soup

Ingredients:
- 2 tablespoons extra virgin olive oil
- 1 small red onion, minced
- 1 medium carrot, peeled and thinly sliced
- 1 celery rib, thinly sliced
- 5 garlic cloves finely minced
- 1 teaspoon Hungarian paprika
- 2 cups vegetable stock
- 1/4 cup wine vinegar

Directions:
1. Heat the oil over medium-high heat.
2. Sauté red onions until tender for about 5 minutes.
3. Slowly add carrots, celery, garlic cloves and Hungarian paprika Cook for another 5 minutes, or until carrots become tender.
4. Add vegetable broth and vinegar Boil and simmer. Cook for 15 minutes longer.

French Red Soup

Ingredients:

- 2 tablespoons olive oil
- 2 large red onions, minced
- 1 small turnip, peeled and thinly sliced
- 1 celery rib, thinly sliced
- 1/2 teaspoon herbes de Provence
- 1 cup vegetable stock
- 1 cup vegetable broth
- 1/4 cup wine vinegar

Directions:

1. Heat the oil over medium-high heat.
2. Sauté red onions until tender for about 5 minutes.
3. Slowly add turnip, celery, and herbs de Provence
4. Cook for another 5 minutes, or until the turnip becomes tender.
5. Add vegetable broth, stock and vinegar.
6. Boil and simmer.
7. Cook for 15 minutes longer.

Thai Roasted Spicy Black Beans and Choy Sum

Ingredients:
- cooking spray
- 1 tablespoon sesame oil
- 3 cloves garlic, minced
- 1/2 teaspoon sea salt
- 1 tbsp. Thai chili paste
- 1/4 teaspoon ground black pepper
- 3 1/2 cups Choy Sum, coarsely chopped
- 2 1/2 cups cherry tomatoes
- 1 (15 ounce) can black beans, drained
- 1 lime, cut into wedges
- 1 tablespoon chopped fresh cilantro

Directions:
1. Preheat your oven to 450 degrees F.
2. Line a baking sheet with foil and grease with sesame oil.
3. Mix the olive oil, garlic, salt, Thai chili paste, and pepper in a bowl.
4. Add in the choy sum, tomatoes, and black beans.
5. Combine until well coated.
6. Spread them out in a single layer on the baking sheet.
7. Add the lime wedges.

8. Roast in the oven until vegetables become caramelized, for about 25 minutes.
9. Take out the lime wedges and top with the cilantro.

ROASTED VEGETABLES

Simple Roasted Broccoli and Cauliflower

Ingredients:
- cooking spray
- 1 tablespoon extra virgin olive oil
- 3 cloves garlic, minced
- 1/2 teaspoon sea salt
- 1/4 teaspoon ground black pepper
- 3 1/2 cups broccoli florets
- 2 1/2 cups cauliflower florets
- 1 tablespoon chopped fresh thyme

Directions:
1. Preheat your oven to 450 degrees F.
2. Line a baking sheet with foil and grease with olive oil.
3. Mix the olive oil, garlic, salt, and pepper in a bowl.
4. Add in the cauliflower and tomatoes.
5. Combine until well coated. Spread them out in a single layer on the baking sheet.
6. Roast in the oven until vegetables become caramelized, for about 25 minutes.
7. Top with the thyme.
8. Simple

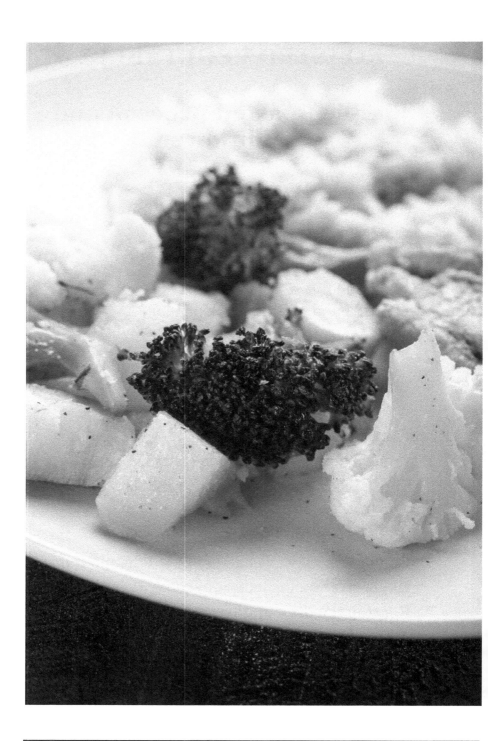

Roasted Spinach and Mustard Greens Extra

Ingredients:
- cooking spray
- 1 tablespoon extra virgin olive oil
- 1/2 teaspoon sea salt
- 1/4 teaspoon ground black pepper

Main Ingredients:
- 1 bunch of mustard greens, rinsed and drained
- 1 bunch of spinach, rinsed and drained

Directions:
1. Preheat your oven to 450 degrees F.
2. Line a baking sheet with foil and grease with olive oil.
3. Mix the extra ingredients thoroughly.
4. Add in the main ingredients.
5. Combine until well coated.
6. Spread them out in a single layer on the baking sheet.
7. Roast in the oven until vegetables become caramelized, for about 25 minutes.

Roasted Napa Cabbage and Turnips Extra

Ingredients:
- cooking spray
- 1 tablespoon extra virgin olive oil
- 1/2 teaspoon sea salt
- 1/4 teaspoon ground black pepper

Main Ingredients:
- 1/2 medium Napa cabbage, sliced thinly
- 1 medium turnip, sliced thinly

Directions:
1. Preheat your oven to 450 degrees F.
2. Line a baking sheet with foil and grease with olive oil
3. Mix the extra ingredients thoroughly.
4. Add in the main ingredients.
5. Combine until well coated.
6. Spread them out in a single layer on the baking sheet.
7. Roast in the oven until vegetables become caramelized, for about 25 minutes.

Simple Roasted

Kale Artichoke Heart and Choy Sum Extra

Ingredients:
- cooking spray
- 1 tablespoon extra virgin olive oil
- 1/2 teaspoon sea salt
- 1/4 teaspoon ground black pepper

Main Ingredients:
- 1 bunch of kale, rinsed and drained
- 1 cup canned artichoke hearts
- 1/2 medium Chinese flowery cabbage (choy sum), coarsely chopped

Directions:
1. Preheat your oven to 450 degrees F.
2. Line a baking sheet with foil and grease with olive oil.
3. Mix the extra ingredients thoroughly.
4. Add in the main ingredients.
5. Combine until well coated.
6. Spread them out in a single layer on the baking sheet.
7. Roast in the oven until vegetables become caramelized, for about 25 minutes

Roasted Spinach and Mustard Greens Extra

Ingredients:
- cooking spray
- 1 tablespoon extra virgin olive oil
- 1/2 teaspoon sea salt
- 1/4 teaspoon ground black pepper

Main Ingredients:
- 5 baby carrots
- 1 bunch of spinach, rinsed and drained
- 1 bunch of mustard greens, rinsed and drained

Directions:
1. Preheat your oven to 450 degrees F.
2. Line a baking sheet with foil and grease with olive oil.
3. Mix the extra ingredients thoroughly.
4. Add in the main ingredients.
5. Combine until well coated.
6. Spread them out in a single layer on the baking sheet.
7. Roast in the oven until vegetables become caramelized, for about 25 minutes.

Roasted Kale and Bok Choy Extra

Ingredients:
- cooking spray
- 1 tablespoon extra virgin olive oil
- 1/2 teaspoon sea salt
- 1/4 teaspoon ground black pepper

Main Ingredients:
- 1 bunch of kale, rinsed and drained
- 1 bunch of bok choy, rinsed ,drained and coarsely chopped

Directions:
1. Preheat your oven to 450 degrees F.
2. Line a baking sheet with foil and grease with olive oil.
3. Mix the extra ingredients thoroughly.
4. Add in the main ingredients.
5. Combine until well coated.
6. Spread them out in a single layer on the baking sheet.
7. Roast in the oven until vegetables become caramelized, for about 25 minutes.

Roasted Lima Beans and Summer Squash

Ingredients:
- 2 (15 ounce) cans lima beans, rinsed and drained
- 1/2 summer squash - peeled, seeded, and cut into 1-inch pieces
- 1 red onion, diced
- 1 sweet potato, peeled and cut into 1-inch cubes
- 2 large carrots, cut into 1 inch pieces
- 3 medium potatoes, cut into 1-inch pieces
- 3 tablespoons sesame oil

Seasoning ingredients:
- 1 teaspoon salt
- 1/2 teaspoon ground black pepper
- 1 teaspoon onion powder
- 2 teaspoon garlic powder
- 1 teaspoon ground fennel seeds
- 1 teaspoon dried rubbed sage

Garnishing Ingredients:
- 2 green onions, chopped (optional)

Directions:
1. Preheat your oven to 350 degrees F.
2. Grease your baking pan.

3. Combine the beans, summer squash, onion, sweet potato, carrots, and russet potatoes on the prepared sheet pan.
4. Drizzle with the oil and toss to coat.
5. Combine the seasoning ingredients in a bowl.
6. Sprinkle them over the vegetables on the pan and toss to coat with seasonings.
7. Bake in the oven for 25 minutes.
8. Stir frequently until vegetables are soft and lightly browned and beans are crisp, for about 20 to 25 minutes more.
9. Season with more salt and black pepper to taste, top with the green onion before serving.

Roasted Soy Beans and Winter Squash

Ingredients:
- 2 (15 ounce) cans soybeans, rinsed and drained
- 1/2 winter squash - peeled, seeded, and cut into 1-inch pieces
- 1 red onion, diced
- 1 sweet potato, peeled and cut into 1-inch cubes
- 2 large carrots, cut into 1 inch pieces
- 3 medium potatoes, cut into 1-inch pieces
- 4 tablespoons extra virgin oil

Seasoning ingredients:
- 1 teaspoon salt
- 1/2 teaspoon ground black pepper
- 1 teaspoon onion powder
- 1 teaspoon dried basil
- 1 teaspoon Italian seasoning

Garnishing Ingredients:
- 2 green onions, chopped (optional)

Directions:
1. Preheat your oven to 350 degrees F.
2. Grease your baking pan.
3. Combine the beans, squash, onion, sweet potato, carrots, and russet potatoes on the prepared sheet pan.

4. Drizzle with the oil and toss to coat.
5. Combine the seasoning ingredients in a bowl.
6. Sprinkle them over the vegetables on the pan and toss to coat with seasonings.
7. Bake in the oven for 25 minutes.
8. Stir frequently until vegetables are soft and lightly browned and beans are crisp, for about 20 to 25 minutes more.
9. Season with more salt and black pepper to taste, top with the green onion before serving.

Chinese Roasted Button Mushrooms and Butternut Squash

Ingredients:
- 2 (15 ounce) cans button mushrooms, sliced and drained
- 1/2 butternut squash - peeled, seeded, and cut into 1-inch pieces
- 1 red onion, diced
- 2 large carrots, cut into 1 inch pieces
- 3 medium turnips, cut into 1-inch pieces
- 3 tablespoons sesame oil

Seasoning ingredients:
- 1 teaspoon salt
- 1/2 teaspoon ground black pepper
- 1 teaspoon onion powder
- 2 teaspoon garlic powder
- 1 teaspoon Sichuan peppercorns
- 1 teaspoon Chinese five-spice powder

Garnishing Ingredients:
- 2 green onions, chopped (optional)

Directions:
1. Preheat your oven to 350 degrees F.
2. Grease your baking pan.
3. Combine the main ingredients on the prepared sheet pan.
4. Drizzle with the oil and toss to coat.

5. Combine the seasoning ingredients in a bowl.
6. Sprinkle them over the vegetables on the pan and toss to coat with seasonings.
7. Bake in the oven for 25 minutes.
8. Stir frequently until vegetables are soft and lightly browned and chickpeas are crisp, for about 20 to 25 minutes more.
9. Season with more salt and black pepper to taste, top with the green onion before serving.

Roasted Button Mushrooms and Squash

Ingredients:
- 2 (15 ounce) cans button mushrooms, rinsed and drained
- 1/2 summer squash - peeled, seeded, and cut into 1-inch pieces
- 1 red onion, diced
- 2 large turnips, cut into 1 inch pieces
- 2 large parsnips, cut into 1 inch pieces
- 3 medium potatoes, cut into 1-inch pieces
- 3 tablespoons butter

Seasoning ingredients:
- 1 teaspoon salt
- 1/2 teaspoon ground black pepper
- 1 teaspoon onion powder
- 2 teaspoon garlic powder
- 1 teaspoon Herbes de Provence

Garnishing Ingredients:
- 2 sprigs of thyme, chopped (optional)

Directions:
1. Preheat your oven to 350 degrees F.
2. Grease your baking pan.
3. Combine the main ingredients on the prepared sheet pan.

4. Drizzle with the melted butter or margarine and toss to coat.
5. Combine the seasoning ingredients in a bowl.
6. Sprinkle them over the vegetables on the pan and toss to coat with seasonings.
7. Bake in the oven for 25 minutes.
8. Stir frequently until vegetables are soft and lightly browned and chickpeas are crisp, for about 20 to 25 minutes more.
9. Season with more salt and black pepper to taste, top with thyme before serving.

MAIN COURSES

Simple Red Bean and Jalapeno Burrito

Ingredients:
- 2 (10 inch) flour tortillas
- 2 tablespoons olive oil
- 1 small red onion, chopped
- 1/2 green bell pepper, chopped
- 2 teaspoon minced garlic
- 1 (15 ounce) can red beans, rinsed and drained
- 1 teaspoon minced jalapeno peppers
- 3 ounces ricotta cheese
- 1/2 teaspoon sea salt
- 2 tablespoons chopped fresh cilantro
- Wrap tortillas in a foil.
- Bake them in a preheated 350 degree oven for 15 minutes.

Directions:
1. Heat oil in a pan over medium heat.
2. Place red onion, bell pepper, garlic and jalapenos in a pan.
3. Cook for 2 minutes while stirring occasionally.
4. Pour the beans into the pan and cook for 3 minutes while constantly stirring.

5. Cut dairy free cream cheese into cubes and add to the pan with salt.
6. Cook for 2 minutes while stirring.
7. Add cilantro into this mixture.
8. Spoon this evenly on the center of every warmed tortilla and roll the tortillas up.

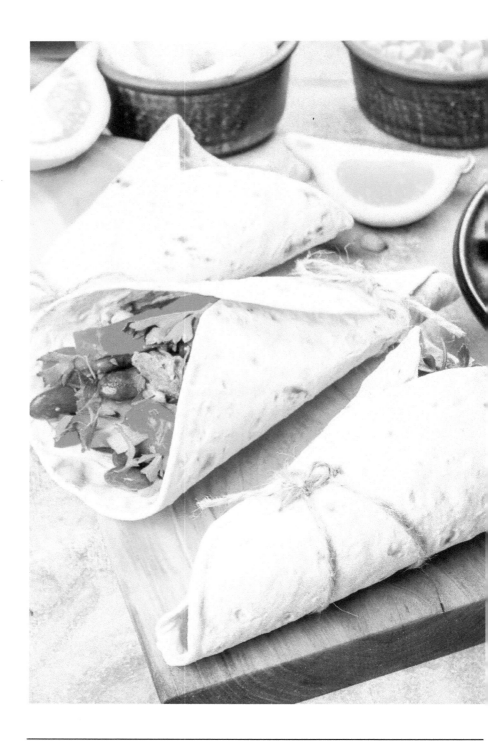

Ramen and Tofu Stir Fry with Sweet and Sour Sauce

Ingredients:
- 1 (3.5 ounce) package ramen noodles (such as Nissin(R) Top Ramen)
- 3 tablespoons sesame seed oil
- 1 slice firm tofu, cubed
- 1/2 thai bird chillies, chopped
- 1/4 small red onion, chopped
- 1/3 cup plum sauce
- 1/3 cup sweet and sour sauce

Directions:
1. Boil a pot of lightly salted water.
2. Cook the noodles in boiling water and stir occasionally, until noodles are tender but still firm to the bite, 2 to 3 minutes.
3. Drain the noodles. Heat oil in a pan over high heat.
4. Place the tofu on one side of the pan.
5. Place the chilies and the red onion on the other side of the pan.
6. Cook a tofu until browned on all sides for 2 minutes.
7. Cook and stir onion and pepper until browned, 2 minutes.
8. Stir in the noodles into the pan.
9. Combine the noodles, tofu, onion, and pepper.

10. Pour the plum sauce and sweet and sour sauce over the noodles.
11. Sauté until well-combined for 3 minutes.

Spicy Curried Purple Cabbage

Ingredients:
- 3 tablespoons olive oil
- 2 dried red chili peppers, broken into pieces
- 2 tsp. skinned split black lentils (urad dal)
- 1 teaspoon split Bengal gram (chana dal)
- 1 teaspoon mustard seed
- 1 sprig fresh curry leaves
- 1 pinch asafoetida powder
- 4 green chili peppers, minced
- 1 head purple cabbage, finely chopped
- 1/4 cup frozen peas (optional) salt to taste
- 1/4 cup grated coconut

Directions:
1. Heat the oil in a pan on medium-high heat.
2. Fry the red peppers, lentils, Bengal gram, and mustard seed in the oil.
3. When the lentils begin to brown, add the curry leaves and asafoetida powder and stir.
4. Add the green chili peppers and cook for a minute more.
5. Combine the cabbage and peas into this mixture.
6. Season with sea salt.
7. Cook until the cabbage wilts, for about 10 minutes.
8. Add the coconut to the mixture and cook for 2 minutes more.

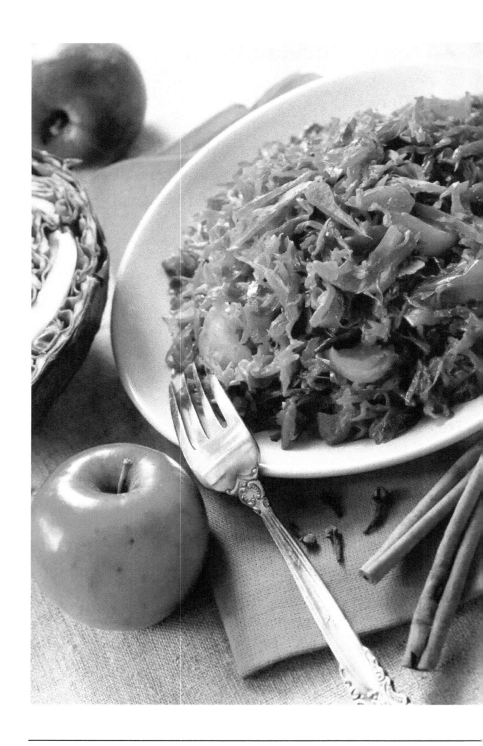

Pesto Zucchini Noodles

Ingredients:
- 1 tablespoon extra virgin olive oil
- 4 small zucchini, cut into noodle-shape strands
- 1/2 cup drained and rinsed chickpeas
- 3 tablespoons pesto, salt and ground black pepper to taste
- 2 tablespoons parmesan cheese
- ¼ cup grated gouda cheese

Directions:
1. Heat olive oil in a pan over medium heat.
2. Cook the zucchini until tender for around 8 minutes.
3. Add the chickpeas and pesto to the zucchini.
4. Lower the heat to medium-low.
5. Cook until the chickpeas are warm and zucchini is coated for about 5 minutes.
6. Season with salt and pepper.
7. Transfer zucchini to a bowl and top with vegan cheese.

Simple Caramelized Carrots

Ingredients:
- 3 tbsp olive (a vegan brand, such as Earth Balance)
- 4 carrots (sliced into ¼ inch thick slices)
- 2 tbsp maple syrup

Directions:
1. Heat the olive oil on low.
2. Add the carrots.
3. Increase the heat to medium-high and add the honey.
4. Let the carrots cook
5. Stir frequently until soft.

Cauliflower and Carrot Stir-fry Batter

Ingredients:
- 1 tablespoon cornstarch
- 1 1/2 cloves garlic, crushed
- 1 teaspoons chopped fresh ginger root, divided
- 1/4 cup olive oil, divided
- 1 small head cauliflower , cut into florets
- 1/2 cup snow peas
- 3/4 cup julienned carrots
- 1/2 cup halved green beans
- 2 tablespoons soy sauce
- 2 1/2 tablespoons water
- 1/4 cup chopped red onion
- 1/2 tablespoon sea salt
- 1 teaspoons chopped fresh ginger root

Directions:
1. In a bowl, combine the batter ingredients and 2 tablespoons olive oil until cornstarch dissolves.
2. Combine the broccoli, snow peas, carrots, and green beans, tossing to lightly coat.
3. Heat remaining 2 tablespoons of oil in a pan over medium heat.
4. Cook vegetables for 2 minutes Add the soy sauce and water.
5. Add the onion, salt, and remaining 1 teaspoon ginger.

6. Cook until vegetables are tender but still crisp.

Roasted Winter Squash

Ingredients:

- One 3-pound winter squash-peeled, seeded and cut into 1-inch dice
- 2 tablespoons extra-virgin olive oil 1 1/2 teaspoons ground cumin
- 1 teaspoon ground parsley
- 1/4 teaspoon cayenne pepper
- Kosher salt and freshly ground pepper

Directions:

1. Preheat your oven to 425°.
2. In a bowl, combine the squash with the olive oil, cumin, coriander and cayenne.
3. Season with salt and pepper.
4. Layer the squash on a baking pan.
5. Roast in your oven for about 40 minutes or until tender

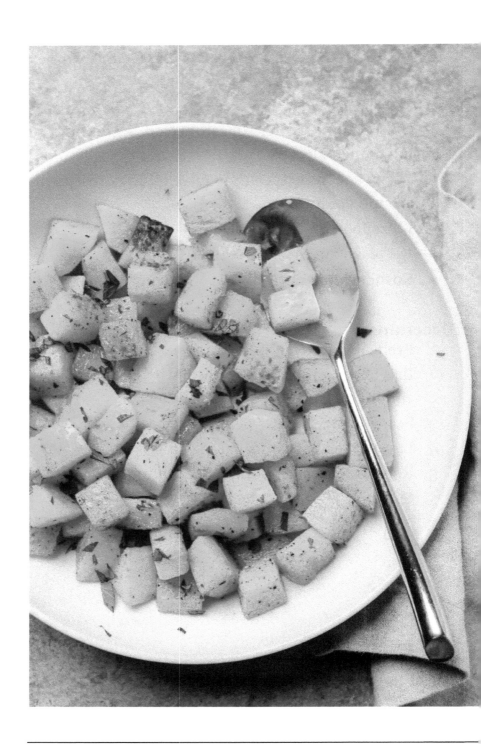

Baked Summer Squash and Red Bell Peppers

Ingredients:
- 1 small summer squash, cubed
- 2 red bell peppers, seeded and diced
- 1 sweet potato, peeled and cubed
- 3 Yukon Gold potatoes, cubed
- 1 red onion, quartered
- 1 tablespoon chopped fresh thyme
- 2 tablespoons chopped fresh rosemary
- 1/4 cup extra virgin olive oil
- 2 tablespoons balsamic vinegar Sea salt
- Freshly ground black pepper

Directions:
1. Preheat your oven to 475 degrees F.
2. Combine the squash, red bell peppers, sweet potato, and potatoes thoroughly.
3. Separate the red onion quarters and add them.
4. Combine the thyme, rosemary, olive oil, vinegar, salt, and pepper.
5. Toss this together with vegetables.
6. Layer on a large roasting pan.
7. Roast for 38 minutes in the oven, while stirring every 10 minutes, or until vegetables start to brown.

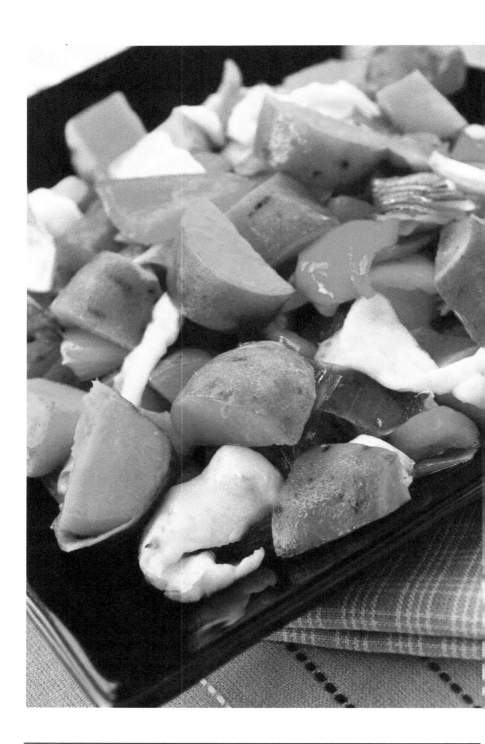

Vegetarian Enchilada

Ingredients:
- 1 Tbsp canola oil
- 1 1/4 cups chopped red onion (1 medium)
- 1 1/4 cups chopped green bell pepper (1 medium)
- 5 cloves garlic, minced
- 1 1/2 cups dry quinoa
- 2 1/4 cups vegetable stock
- 1 (14.5 oz) can tomatoes with green chilies, not drained
- 1 8 oz can tomato sauce
- 2 Tbsp. chili powder
- 1 1/2 tsp ground cumin
- Salt and freshly ground black pepper, to taste
- 1 (14.5 oz) can black beans, drained and rinsed
- 1 (14.5 oz) can pinto beans, drained and rinsed
- 1 1/2 cups frozen corn
- 1 1/2 cups gouda cheese , shredded
- Sea salt
- Black pepper

Toppings:
- Diced avocados , diced Roma tomatoes, chopped cilantro, lime wedges, chopped green onions

Directions:
1. Heat oil in a pan over medium.

2. In this oiled pan, sauté onion and bell pepper for 3 minutes.
3. Add in the garlic and sauté 30 seconds longer.
4. Pour the contents of the pan into a slow cooker.
5. Cover and cook on high for 3 hours,
6. Add the corn and beans.
7. Combine well and top with vegan cheese.
8. Cover and cook for 13 minutes longer.

Slow Cooked Macaroni and Vegan Cheese

Ingredients:

- 1 red onion, medium chopped
- 1 green bell pepper chopped
- 15 ounce can black beans rinsed and drained
- 15 ounce can garbanzo beans rinsed and drained
- 28 ounce crushed tomatoes
- 1 ½ tablespoons chili powder
- 2 teaspoons cumin
- ½ teaspoon salt
- 1/8 teaspoon black pepper
- 2 cups vegetable stock
- 8 ounces whole wheat elbow macaroni pasta uncooked
- 1 ½ cups Vegan Cheese (Tofu Based)
- chopped green onions for serving

Directions:

1. Put all of the ingredients except for pasta, vegan cheese, and green onions in your slow cooker.
2. Combine and cover.
3. Cook on high heat for 4 hours or low heat for 7 hours.
4. Add the pasta and cook on high heat for 18 minutes, or until pasta becomes al dente.
5. Add 1 cup of cheese and stir.
6. Garnish with the remaining vegan cheese and green onions

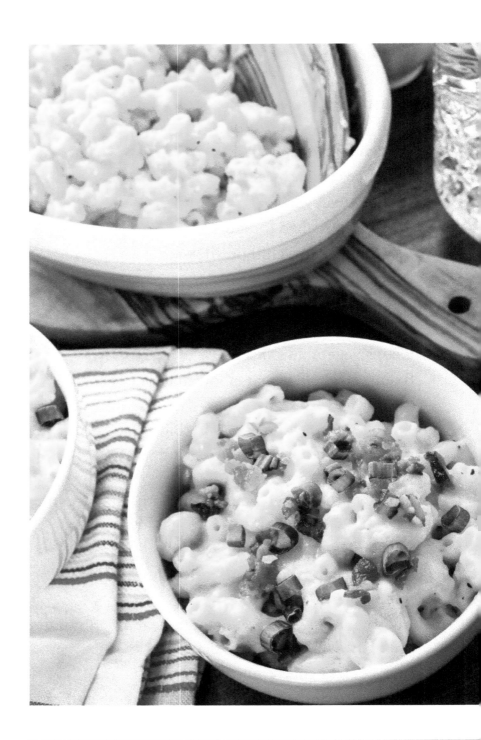

Fettuccini and Pesto

Ingredients:
- 15 ounce can kidney beans
- 15 ounce can black beans
- 28 ounce crushed tomatoes
- 4 tbsp. pesto
- 1 tsp. Italian seasoning
- ½ teaspoon salt
- 1/8 teaspoon black pepper
- 2 cups vegetable stock
- 8 ounces fettuccini uncooked
- 1 ½ cups Vegan Cheese (Tofu Based)

Garnishing :
- chopped green onions for serving

Directions:
1. Put all of the ingredients except for pasta, vegan cheese, and garnishing ingredients in your slow cooker.
2. Combine and cover.
3. Cook on high heat for 4 hours or low heat for 7 hours.
4. Add the pasta and cook on high heat for 18 minutes, or until pasta becomes al dente.
5. Add 1 cup of cheese and stir.
6. Sprinkle with the remaining vegan cheese and garnishing ingredients

SALADS

Marinated Roasted Beets and Pecans Salad

Ingredients:
- 6 medium beets, cooked and quartered
- 6 cups fresh arugula
- 1/2 cup pecans, toasted, coarsely chopped
- 1/4 cup dried cherries 1/2 avocado, peeled, pitted, and cubed
- 2 ounces brie cheese, crumbled
- 2 ounces cheddar cheese , shredded

Dressing:
- 1/4 cup balsamic vinegar
- 3 tablespoons leeks, thinly sliced
- 4 tsp. honey
- 1/3 cup extra-virgin olive oil
- Salt and freshly ground black pepper

Directions:
1. Preheat the oven to 450 degrees F.
2. Combine all of the dressing ingredients except the olive oil in a food processor.
3. Slowly pour in the olive oil.
4. Coat the beets with the dressing and place on a greased cookie sheet.

5. Roast while flipping every 3-4 min. for a total of 13 min. or until caramelized.
6. Let it cool down.
7. Toss the rest of the ingredients together.

Couscous with Blue Cheese Salad

Ingredients:
- 1 box flavored couscous (garlic or Parmesan), cooked
- 1 can chickpeas
- 1 green bell pepper, finely chopped
- 1/2 Vidalia onion, chopped
- 1 cucumber, peeled, seeded, and finely chopped
- 3 plum tomatoes, chopped
- 2 ounces camembert cheese, crumbled
- 2 ounces brie cheese, crumbled
- 1/2 cup crumbled soft goat cheese
- Salt and freshly ground black pepper
- 1/4 cup olive oil
- 1-2 lemons, juiced

Directions:
1. Toss all of the ingredients together and combine well.

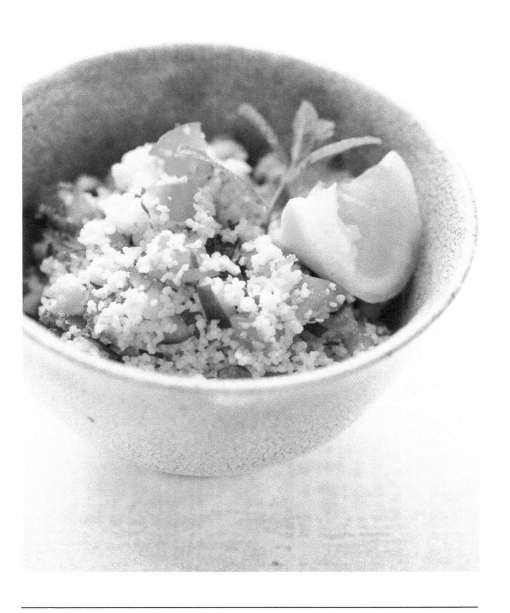

Marinated Tomato with Pecorino Romano Salad

Ingredients:

- 3 tablespoons chopped fresh parsley leaves
- 1 tablespoon honey
- 1 1/2 teaspoons garlic salt
- 1 1/2 teaspoons seasoned salt
- 2 ounces pecorino romano cheese, shredded
- 1 ounce monterey jack cheese, shredded
- 3/4 cup olive oil
- 1/2 cup white wine vinegar
- 2 to 3 green onions, chopped
- 4 to 6 large tomatoes, each cut into 6 wedges

Directions:

1. Combine all of the ingredients except the tomatoes.
2. Whisk and combine well.
3. Marinate the tomatoes with this mixture inside a resealable plastic bag for 2 hours while turning the bag every hour.

Corn Beans and Cottage Cheese

Ingredients:

- 2 ears fresh corn or 1 cup frozen corn, thawed
- 1 (15-ounce) can red kidney beans, drained and rinsed
- 1 (15-ounce) can garbanzo beans, drained and rinsed
- 1 green bell pepper, cored, seeded, and cut into 1/2-inch pieces
- 1 mango, peeled, seeded, and cut into 1/2-inch pieces
- 2 ounces cottage cheese, crumbled
- 2 ounces feta cheese, crumbled

Dressing:

- 1 lemon, zested and juiced
- 2 tablespoons balsamic vinegar
- 1/2 cup chopped fresh basil leaves
- ½ teaspoon chili powder
- 1/3 cup extra-virgin olive oil Kosher salt and freshly ground black pepper

Directions:

1. Combine all of the dressing ingredients except the oil.
2. Slowly drizzle the oil into the dressing mixture.
3. Preheat the grill.
4. Peel back the corn husks and soak in cold water for 30 min.
5. Drain and grill for 12 min.

6. Remove the husk and let it cool down.
7. Remove the kernels and combine the rest of the remaining ingredients except the dressing mixture with the corn.
8. Toss all of the ingredients together.

Melon and Ricotta Salad

Ingredients:
- 1 (5-pound) watermelon, cut into bite sized pieces and deseed
- 1 sweet onion, peeled and sliced into rings
- 4 ounces vegan cheese, crumbled
- 2 tablespoons chopped fresh mint
- 2 ounces pepper jack cheese, shredded
- 2 ounces ricotta cheese

Dressing:
- 1/4 cup white wine vinegar
- Salt and pepper
- 1/2 cup extra-virgin olive oil

Directions:
1. Combine all of the dressing ingredients together in a food processor.
2. Toss all of the ingredients together.

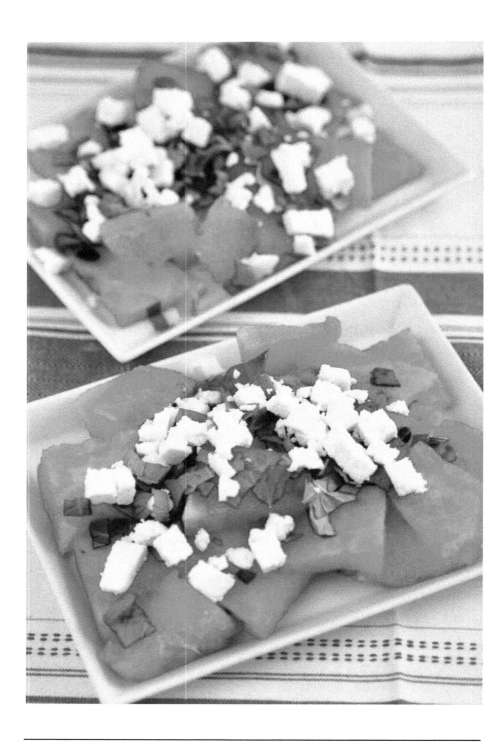

Asparagus Cream Cheese and Pecan Salad

Ingredients:

- 1/2 pound Asparagus spears, trimmed
- 2 tablespoons chopped pecan
- 2 tablespoons finely chopped fresh parsley leaves
- 2 tablespoons chopped red onion
- 2 teaspoons walnut oil
- 2 ounces cream cheese, crumbled

Dressing:

- 1 teaspoon red wine
- 1 teaspoon vinegar
- English mustard
- Salt and pepper

Directions:

1. Bring a large pot of water to a boil and steam the asparagus.
2. Let it cool down.
3. Toast the pecans in medium heat until fragrant and let it cool down.
4. Combine all of the dressing ingredients.
5. Toss all of the ingredients together.

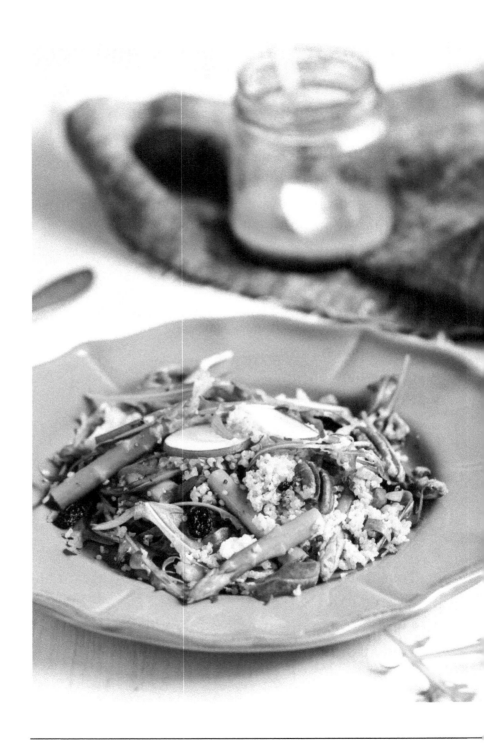

San Marzano Tomatoes with Balsamic Reduction Dressing

Ingredients:
- 1 cup balsamic vinegar
- 1 cup pitted green olives, halved
- 1/4 cup chopped fresh parsley leaves
- 2 tablespoons capers, rinsed and drained
- ½ tsp. garlic powder
- 8 fresh basil leaves, shredded
- 1/2 teaspoon freshly ground assorted peppercorns
- 6 tablespoons extra-virgin olive oil
- 1 pound ripe San Marzano tomatoes
- 2 ounces gouda cheese, shredded

Directions:
1. Cook the balsamic vinegar over low heat for 20 min. or until thick.
2. Combine the olives, parsley, anchovies, capers, garlic powder, basil, peppercorns and olive oil.
3. Slice the tomatoes into ¼-inch rounds and place on a plate.
4. Spoon the olives and parsley over the tomatoes.
5. Drizzle with the balsamic reduction sauce.
6. Garnish with mint.

Japanese Noodle Salad

Ingredients:

- 1 package soba noodles
- 1 parsnip, thinly sliced or julienned
- 2 celery stalks, thinly sliced or julienned
- 5 green onions, bottom 4 inches, thinly sliced
- 1/2 cup thinly sliced red cabbage
- 1/2 green bell pepper, thinly sliced or julienned
- 1/2 cup julienned bok choy
- 3 tablespoons minced fresh cilantro leaves
- 2 ounces pecorino romano cheese, shredded

Dressing:

- 1 teaspoon sesame oil
- 2 tablespoons dry sherry
- 3 tablespoons soy sauce
- 1 teaspoon hot chili oil
- 1 tablespoon hoisin sauce
- 5 tablespoons extra-virgin olive oil

Directions:

1. Bring salted water to a boil and add the soba noodles.
2. Cook until tender. Place the noodles in an ice bath and drain.
3. Combine all of the dressing ingredients.
4. In a separate bowl, combine the rest of the ingredients except the peanuts and sesame seeds.
5. Combine all of the ingredients except the peanuts and sesame seeds and toss.

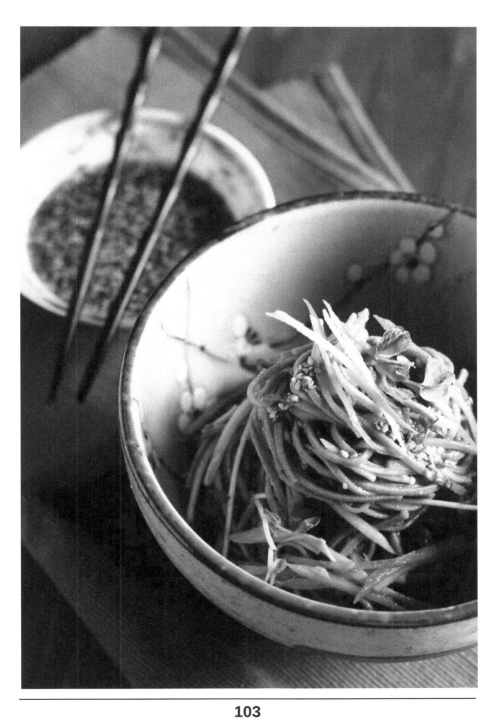

Watercress and Celeriac Bulb Salad

Ingredients:
- 3 bunches watercress, washed thoroughly and spun on the salad spinner
- 2 ounces cottage cheese, crumbled
- 2 ounces feta cheese, crumbled
- 1 celeriac bulb, peeled and grated (do this right before serving so it doesn't oxidize and turn brown)
- Kosher salt and freshly ground black pepper

Dressing:
- 1/2 cup shelled almonds, plus more for garnish
- 1/2 tsp. garlic powder
- 4 tbsp. apple cider vinegar
- 1/2 teaspoon honey
- About 1/2 cup hot water
- Sea salt and freshly ground black pepper
- 1/2 cup extra virgin olive oil
- Splash good extra-virgin olive oil, for dressing

Directions:
1. Toast the nuts in a skillet and stir frequently until you smell an aroma and set aside.
2. In a blender combine all of the ingredients until smooth while adding water if needed.
3. In a separate bowl, combine the rest of the ingredients.
4. Combine all of the ingredients together and toss.

Bib Lettuce and Celeriac Bulb Salad

Ingredients:
- 3 bunches Bib Lettuce , washed thoroughly and spun on the salad spinner.
- 2 ounces gouda cheese, shredded
- 2 ounces pecorino romano cheese, shredded
- 1 celeriac bulb, peeled and grated (do this right before serving so it doesn't oxidize and turn brown)
- Kosher salt and freshly ground black pepper

Dressing:
- 1/2 cup cashew nuts, plus more for garnish
- 1/2 tsp. garlic powder
- 1 tsp. lime juice
- 1/2 teaspoon cayenne pepper
- About 1/2 cup hot water
- Kosher salt and freshly ground black pepper
- 1/2 cup extra virgin olive oil
- Splash good extra-virgin olive oil, for dressing

Directions:
1. Toast the nuts in a skillet and stir frequently until you smell an aroma and set aside.
2. In a blender combine all of the ingredients until smooth while adding water if needed.
3. In a separate bowl, combine the rest of the ingredients.
4. Combine all of the ingredients together and toss.

Watercress Mango and Brie Cheese Salad

Ingredients:
- 3 bunches watercress, washed thoroughly and spun on the salad spinner
- 1 mango, cored and cubed
- 2 ounces brie cheese, crumbled
- 2 ounces cheddar cheese , shredded
- Kosher salt and freshly ground black pepper

Dressing:
- 1/2 cup shelled walnuts, plus more for garnish
- 1/2 tsp. garlic powder
- 4 tbsp. vinegar
- 1/2 teaspoon chili garlic paste
- About 1/2 cup hot water Kosher salt and freshly ground black pepper
- 1/2 cup sesame oil Splash good sesame oil, for dressing

Directions:
1. Toast the nuts in a skillet and stir frequently until you smell an aroma and set aside.
2. In a blender combine all of the ingredients until smooth while adding water if needed.
3. In a separate bowl, combine the rest of the ingredients.
4. Combine all of the ingredients together and toss.

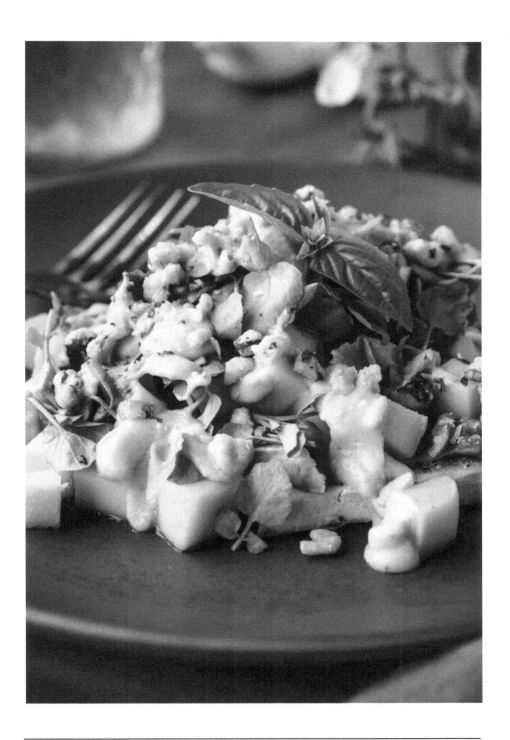

Bib Lettuce Celeriac Bulb and Feta Cheese Salad

Ingredients:
- 3 bunches Bib Lettuce , washed thoroughly and spun on the salad spinner
- 2 ounces cottage cheese, crumbled
- 2 ounces feta cheese, crumbled
- 1 celeriac bulb, peeled and grated (do this right before serving so it doesn't oxidize and turn brown)
- Kosher salt and freshly ground black pepper

Dressing:
- 1/2 cup shelled almonds, plus more for garnish
- 1/2 tsp. garlic powder
- 4 tbsp. apple cider vinegar
- 1/2 teaspoon honey
- About 1/2 cup hot water
- Sea salt and freshly ground black pepper
- 1/2 cup extra virgin olive oil
- Splash good extra-virgin olive oil, for dressing

Directions:
1. Toast the nuts in a skillet and stir frequently until you smell an aroma and set aside.
2. In a blender combine all of the ingredients until smooth while adding water if needed.
3. In a separate bowl, combine the rest of the ingredients.
4. Combine all of the ingredients together and toss.

Notes